CW00406601

THE GLUCOSE REVOLUTION

Understanding the Importance of Blood Sugar Management

By

Noah Keaton

Copyright © by Noah Keaton 2023.

All rights reserved.
Before this document is duplicated or reproduced in any manner, the publisher's consent must be gained. Therefore, the contents within can neither be stored electronically, transferred, nor kept in a database. Neither in Part nor full can the document be copied, scanned, faxed, or retained without approval from the publisher or creator.

TABLE OF CONTENTS

INTRODUCTION TO THE GLUCOSE REVOLUTION

The Glucose Revolution is a term coined to describe the significant shift in our understanding of carbohydrates and their impact on our health. It represents a change in the way we think about carbohydrates, particularly glucose, and how they affect our bodies. The Glucose Revolution is a book written by Dr. Jennie Brand-Miller, Kaye Foster-Powell, and Dr. Thomas M.S. Wolever, which has had a significant impact on how we approach nutrition and health.

Before the Glucose Revolution, carbohydrates were often viewed as a single entity, and all were treated equally. However, the Glucose Revolution emphasized the importance of the glycemic index, a ranking of how quickly different carbohydrates raise blood sugar levels. This ranking has revolutionized our understanding of carbohydrates and their impact on our health.

The glycemic index is calculated on a scale of 0 to 100, with glucose receiving a score of 100. Foods with a high glycemic index raise blood sugar levels immediately, whereas those with a low glycemic index raise blood sugar levels slowly. This ranking method has created diets emphasizing low glycemic index carbs. This is because meals with a low glycemic index digest and absorb more slowly, resulting in a slower and more constant increase in blood sugar levels.

The Glucose Revolution has had a profound influence on nutrition and health. It has resulted in the Glycemic Index Diet, which focuses on eating carbs with a low glycemic index. This diet has been demonstrated to enhance blood sugar management and reduce weight in diabetics.

One of the Glycemic Index Diet's main advantages is its emphasis on full, unprocessed meals. This indicates that the diet focuses on fruits, vegetables, whole grains, and lean meats, all of which have a low glycemic index. This diet also stresses the need for fibre, which slows carbohydrate absorption and helps to manage blood sugar levels.

Beyond better blood sugar management, the Glycemic Index Diet has been found to provide a variety of health advantages. According to research, this diet may aid with weight reduction, lower the risk of heart disease, and even enhance cognitive performance.

The discovery of low glycemic index sweeteners has been another key influence of the Glucose Revolution. These sweeteners, including xylitol, erythritol, and stevia, have become popular as consumers seek methods to limit their sugar consumption. These sugar substitutes have a lower glycemic index than sugar, which means they slowly boost blood sugar levels.

Ultimately, the Glucose Revolution has changed the face of nutrition and health. This trend has led to a greater knowledge of how various carbohydrates affect our bodies by highlighting the relevance of the glycemic index. It has also resulted in new diets and sweeteners that may help us enhance our health and live a more balanced lifestyle.

In conclusion, the Glucose Revolution has significantly influenced how we approach nutrition and health. We better understand how different carbohydrates affect our bodies by focusing on the glycemic index. As a result, diets and sweeteners that may help us enhance our health and live a more balanced lifestyle have been developed. The Glucose Revolution is a moving target, and it will be intriguing to watch what discoveries and developments emerge from this subject in the coming years.

CHAPTER 1:

UNDERSTANDING GLUCOSE AND ITS ROLE IN THE BODY

Glucose is a basic sugar serving the human body's principal energy source. It is crucial to human existence and participates in several key bodily functions. In this book, we will look at the function of glucose in the body and how it affects our general health.

Glucose is a carbohydrate in various meals, including fruits, vegetables, and grains. Our digestive system breaks down carbs into glucose molecules, which are subsequently taken into circulation. Glucose enters our circulation and goes to our cells, which are needed to power our body.

The body's cells need glucose to create energy, and our bodies cannot operate properly without it. The brain, in particular, needs extensive glucose to operate and consumes around 20% of the body's energy. The brain cannot operate properly without adequate glucose, which may lead to cognitive impairment.

Glucose, in addition to producing energy, is essential for managing our bodies' blood sugar levels. The pancreas generates insulin, a hormone that helps to control the quantity of glucose in circulation. When we consume carbs, insulin is produced, which allows glucose to enter our cells and be utilized for energy. But, if we consume too many carbs, our blood sugar levels might become excessively high, resulting in various health concerns.

Diabetes is one of the most well-known health issues connected with elevated blood sugar levels. Diabetes is a chronic disease in which the body cannot produce or use insulin effectively, resulting in high blood sugar levels. Diabetes, if left untreated, may cause a variety of consequences, including nerve damage, renal damage, and cardiovascular disease.

It's also important to remember that low blood sugar levels may be just as harmful as high blood sugar levels. When our blood sugar levels fall too low, we may experience dizziness, confusion, and even loss of consciousness. This is why keeping blood sugar levels constant throughout the day is critical.

So, how can we ensure that our bodies get enough glucose without experiencing blood sugar spikes or drops? The trick is to eat carbs in moderation and to pick complex carbohydrates that break down and absorb more slowly. Whole grains, veggies, and legumes are examples of complex carbs. These meals offer a consistent supply of glucose, assisting in maintaining stable blood sugar levels throughout the day.

It's also worth noting that although glucose is an essential energy source for the body, it's not the sole. Other nutrients, such as lipids and proteins, may also be used for energy by the body. Glucose, on the other hand, remains the principal energy source for most cells in the body, notably the brain.

In conclusion, glucose is an important nutrient that plays an important part in our general health. It is our bodies' principal energy source and is involved in various vital activities, including blood sugar regulation and cognitive function. By ingesting complex carbs in moderation, we may guarantee that our bodies acquire adequate glucose without suffering blood sugar spikes or decreases.

Understanding the function of glucose in the body allows us to make educated dietary choices and maintain optimum health.

CHAPTER 2:

THE HISTORY OF THE GLUCOSE REVOLUTION

The phrase "Glucose Revolution" was developed in the late 1990s to characterize the growing recognition of the significance of carbs, especially complex carbohydrates, in maintaining a balanced diet. The Glucose Revolution sought to move the emphasis on nutrition away from low-fat diets and toward diets that stressed the significance of carbs in maintaining stable blood sugar levels. This new nutritional strategy was founded on years of scientific study and represented a substantial shift from standard dietary guidelines.

The Glucose Revolution started in the early twentieth century when scientists first began comprehending carbs' significance in the body. The discovery of insulin, a hormone that controls blood sugar levels, in the 1920s changed diabetes therapy. Scientists started to investigate the effects of carbohydrates on the body in more depth by introducing new tools for monitoring blood sugar levels.

The emphasis on nutrition switched in the 1960s and 1970s to limiting fat consumption since it was thought fat was the major cause of heart disease. Nevertheless, fresh evidence appeared in the 1980s and 1990s that questioned this notion. Scientists recognized that the kind of fat ingested was more essential than the quantity and that carbohydrates, especially complex carbs, were critical in maintaining a healthy diet.

Dr Jennie Brand-Miller, a professor of human nutrition at the University of Sydney in Australia, was a crucial contributor to the creation of the Glucose Revolution. Dr Brand-Miller and her colleagues started researching the glycemic index (GI) in the 1980s, measuring how rapidly carbohydrates are digested and absorbed into circulation. They discovered that high GI meals, such as white bread and potatoes, quickly boosted blood sugar levels, but low GI foods, such as whole grains and legumes, were digested more slowly and offered a more sustained energy source.

Dr Brand-Miller and her colleagues presented their results in "The Glucose Revolution," a book published in Australia in 1996. The book became a best-seller, rekindling interest in the importance of carbs in the diet. It also helped to popularize the notion of the glycemic index by demonstrating that not all carbs are created equal.

The Glucose Revolution swiftly gained hold in the United States and Europe, and several publications and recipes promoting a low-GI diet were released. The diet's primary principle was to take slow-digesting carbs and avoid meals that quickly increased blood sugar levels. The diet recommended eating whole grains, vegetables, fruits, and legumes while avoiding processed meals, sugary beverages, and refined carbs.

Although the Glucose Revolution was first contentious, it has recently gained widespread acceptance among scientists. Several studies have demonstrated a low-GI diet to help lower the risk of heart disease, diabetes, and other chronic illnesses. The diet has also been demonstrated to be useful in regulating blood sugar levels in patients with diabetes, and it is currently recommended as a healthy eating pattern by several health organizations.

One of the most important advantages of the Glucose Revolution is that it encourages a more balanced approach to diet. Rather than vilifying a single nutrient, such as fat, it highlights the benefits of eating a diverse range of nutrients, especially complex carbs. It also encourages individuals to think about the quality of their meals rather than just the number of calories or grams of fat.

The Glucose Revolution has evolved in recent years, with a stronger focus on the value of whole foods and plant-based diets. This transition shows an increasing consciousness.

CHAPTER 3:

THE SCIENCE OF BLOOD SUGAR REGULATION

Blood sugar management, or glucose homeostasis, is a complicated process involving a precise balance of hormones and enzymes to ensure the body has a constant energy source. Glucose is the major energy source for the body's cells; therefore, keeping blood sugar levels steady is critical for good health. The science of blood sugar control, including the roles of hormones, enzymes, and dietary variables, will be discussed in this book.

Blood Sugar Regulation: Hormones and Enzymes

Blood sugar levels are principally regulated by two hormones: insulin and glucagon. Insulin is generated by pancreatic beta cells and has the primary purpose of lowering blood sugar levels. As blood sugar levels rise after a meal, insulin is released into the circulation to assist in the transfer of glucose from the blood into the cells. This is known as glucose absorption, which is essential for keeping blood sugar levels consistent.

Glucagon, on the other hand, is generated by pancreatic alpha cells and primarily aims to increase blood sugar levels. When blood sugar levels go too low, the hormone glucagon is released into the circulation, stimulating the liver to release glucose into the bloodstream. This is known as gluconeogenesis, and it aids in maintaining stable blood sugar levels during fasting or exercise.

Cortisol, another hormone generated by the adrenal glands, also functions in blood sugar management. Cortisol is a stress hormone that stimulates gluconeogenesis in the liver, which may raise blood sugar levels. This reaction is vital in times of stress or danger because it gives the body the energy to respond to a threat.

Many enzymes, in addition to hormones, play a role in blood sugar control. Glucose-6-phosphatase is one of these enzymes found mostly in the liver and kidneys. This enzyme aids in converting glycogen, a kind of stored glucose, back into glucose for release into the circulation. Hexokinase, which is present in many tissues and is responsible for the first step in glucose metabolism, is another enzyme. This enzyme aids in converting glucose to glucose-6-

phosphate, which may subsequently be utilized as energy or stored as glycogen.

Blood Sugar Regulation: Dietary Factors

Dietary factors also have an impact on blood sugar regulation. A food's glycemic index (GI) indicates how rapidly it elevates blood sugar levels. High-GI foods, such as white bread and sugary beverages, are quickly digested and absorbed into the circulation, resulting in a spike in blood sugar levels. Low GI foods, on the other hand, such as whole grains and legumes, are absorbed slowly and give a more prolonged supply of energy.

The glycemic load (GL) is another metric that considers the overall quantity of carbohydrates in a meal and its GI. Even though their GI is modest, foods with a high GL, such as a big dish of white rice, may induce a quick spike in blood sugar levels.

Fibre is also an essential dietary element in controlling blood sugar levels. Soluble fibre, which may be found in foods like oats, beans, and fruits, can aid in limiting the absorption of glucose into the circulation, lowering the risk of blood sugar increases. Insoluble fibre, which may be found in foods like whole grains and vegetables, can aid in enhancing satiety and lower total calorie consumption, which can also assist in managing blood sugar levels.

Blood Sugar Regulation: Implications for Health
Keeping stable blood sugar levels is critical for general health since blood sugar swings may impact the body differently. Hyperglycemia, or high blood

sugar levels, may cause various health concerns, including diabetes and heart disease.

CHAPTER 4:

GLYCEMIC INDEX AND GLYCEMIC LOAD: KEY CONCEPTS

The glycemic index (GI) and glycemic load (GL) are two key concepts in nutrition and health. They assist individuals in understanding how various carbs influence blood sugar levels and how these impacts might affect health. In this essay, we will look at these fundamental principles and their health consequences.

Glycemic Index (GI)

The glycemic index measures how rapidly a carbohydrate-rich diet increases blood sugar levels.

Meals with a high GI are quickly digested and absorbed into the circulation, resulting in a fast rise in blood sugar levels. Low GI foods are digested and absorbed more slowly, resulting in a slower and more persistent rise in blood sugar levels.

The GI is calculated on a scale of 0 to 100, with 100 being the GI of pure glucose (a simple sugar). Foods with a GI of 70 or more are considered high, while those with a GI of 55 or below are considered low. Items having a GI of 56 to 69 are considered moderate on the GI scale.

White bread, sugar-sweetened drinks, and candy are examples of high-GI foods. Most fruits and vegetables, whole grains, and legumes are examples of low-GI foods.

For persons with diabetes or other disorders that impair blood sugar balance, a glycemic index is a valuable tool. High GI foods may induce a quick spike in blood sugar levels, which can be troublesome for people struggling to regulate their blood sugar. Eating low-GI meals may assist in creating more stable blood sugar levels.

Conversely, the glycemic index is not a perfect predictor of how a meal will affect blood sugar levels. A food's GI might change based on how it's cooked and what it's eaten with. A high-GI food, for example, may have a lower impact on blood sugar levels when combined with protein or fat than when consumed alone.

Glycemic Load (GL)

Glycemic load considers both the quantity and quality of carbohydrates in food. It is determined by multiplying the glycemic index of a food by the number of carbohydrates in a serving and then dividing by 100.

Because it considers both the quality and quantity of carbohydrates in a food, the glycemic load is a more comprehensive measure than the glycemic index alone. Even if they are not high on the glycemic index, foods with a high glycemic load can cause a rapid increase in blood sugar levels.

White rice, potatoes, and sweetened drinks are all high-glycemic-load foods. Most fruits and vegetables, whole grains, and legumes are examples of low-glycemic-load foods.

The glycemic load, like the glycemic index, is an important tool for patients with diabetes or other illnesses that influence blood sugar homeostasis. Eating foods with a low glycemic load will assist in producing more stable blood sugar levels and may have other health advantages.

Implications for Health

It is critical for general health to keep blood sugar levels steady. Blood sugar fluctuations may have various repercussions on the body, including an increased risk of diabetes, heart disease, and other health issues.

Selecting foods with low glycemic indexes and loads may assist in creating more stable blood sugar levels, which may have health advantages. These foods are often richer in fibre, vitamins, and minerals and may aid in promoting feelings of fullness and reducing total calorie consumption.

Nevertheless, remember that the glycemic index and load are just two aspects to consider when making dietary decisions. Additional aspects include a food's total nutritional density, its

CHAPTER 5:

THE BENEFITS OF A LOW-GLYCEMIC DIET

A low-glycemic diet focuses on foods with a low glycemic index and glycemic load. This diet has been linked to various health advantages, including improved blood sugar management, heart health, and weight reduction.

In this book, we will review the advantages of a low-glycemic diet.

Improved Blood Sugar Control

Improved blood sugar management is one of the primary advantages of a low-glycemic diet. Meals with a high glycemic index may induce a quick rise in blood sugar levels, which can be troublesome for persons who struggle to control their blood sugar. Selecting foods with a low glycemic index and glycemic load will assist in promoting more stable blood sugar levels and may help to minimize blood sugar spikes and crashes.

A low-glycemic diet has been found in many trials to enhance blood sugar management in persons with diabetes. A low-glycemic diet, for example, improved blood sugar management and lowered insulin resistance in persons with type 2 diabetes, according to research published in the American Journal of Clinical Nutrition.

Improved Heart Health

A low-glycemic diet may also be advantageous to cardiovascular health. High-glycemic-index foods have been found to induce inflammation, which is a major cause of heart disease. Eating meals with low glycemic indexes and loads may assist in decreasing inflammation and enhancing heart health.

A low-glycemic diet has been demonstrated in many trials to enhance heart health indicators. For example, research published in the Journal of the American College of Cardiology discovered that a low-glycemic diet lowered cholesterol levels and decreased inflammatory indicators in overweight and obese people.

Weight Loss

A low-glycemic diet may also help with weight reduction. Low glycemic index and glycemic load foods are often richer in fibre, which may increase feelings of fullness and lower total calorie consumption.

A low-glycemic diet has been found in many trials to help weight reduction. For example, research published in the Journal of the American Medical Association discovered that a low-glycemic diet was more beneficial than a low-fat diet for weight reduction in overweight and obese people.

Other Health Benefits

Apart from the advantages described above, a low-glycemic diet has been linked to several additional health benefits.

As an example:

Better digestion: Foods with a low glycemic index and glycemic load tend to be richer in fibre, which may aid in promoting regular bowel motions and digestion.

Reduced risk of certain cancers: A low-glycemic diet has been linked to a lower risk of certain malignancies, such as breast and colorectal cancer.

Improved cognitive function: A low-glycemic diet has been found to enhance cognitive performance and lower the risk of cognitive decline in older persons.

Tips for Following a Low-Glycemic Diet

If you're interested in following a low-glycemic diet, here are some tips to get you started:

- Eat unprocessed, minimally processed meals: Highly processed foods have a higher glycemic index and load. Select whole foods such as fruits and vegetables, whole grains, and lean protein.

- Choose low-glycemic fruits and veggies: Although most fruits and vegetables have a low glycemic index, some have a lower glycemic index than others. For example, berries, apples, and leafy greens are all excellent alternatives.

- Eat high-glycemic meals with protein or fat: If you prefer to consume foods with a higher glycemic index, eating them with protein or fat may help to decrease their absorption and lessen their influence on blood sugar levels.

- Examine food labels

CHAPTER 6:

FOODS TO AVOID ON A LOW-GLYCEMIC DIET

It is important to be aware of the items high on the glycemic index and should be avoided or restricted while following a low-glycemic diet. Certain meals may produce blood sugar spikes, making it harder to maintain stable blood sugar levels throughout the day. This book will look at some things to avoid on a low-glycemic diet.

Highly Processed Foods

Heavily processed foods have a high glycemic index and should be avoided following a low-glycemic diet. These meals often include added sugars and processed carbs, which may trigger blood sugar increases.

Examples of highly processed foods to avoid include:

- Candy
- Soda
- Cookies and other baked goods
- Chips and other snack foods
- White bread and other refined grains

Instead, prioritize nutritious, minimally processed meals with naturally low glycemic indexes, such as fruits, vegetables, whole grains, and lean protein sources.

Sweetened Beverages

Sweetened beverages are a significant source of added sugars in the American diet and should be avoided following a low-glycemic diet. Drinking drinks may produce abrupt rises in blood sugar levels, leading to insulin resistance and other health concerns in the long run.

Examples of sweetened beverages to avoid include:
- Soda
- Sweetened tea and coffee
- Sports drinks
- Fruit juice

Instead, drink unsweetened tea or coffee or sparkling water flavoured with a piece of lemon or lime.

High-Sugar Fruits

Although most fruits have a low glycemic index, some have a higher glycemic index than others and should be avoided on a low-glycemic diet. These fruits have higher natural sugars and might cause a faster rise in blood sugar levels.

Examples of high-sugar fruits to limit include:

- Pineapple
- Mango
- Bananas
- Grapes
- Dried fruit

Instead, choose lower-sugar fruits like berries, apples, pears, and citrus.

Starchy Vegetables

Starchy vegetables with a high glycemic index, such as potatoes and maize, should be avoided on a low-glycemic diet. These veggies contain more carbs than non-starchy vegetables and may cause blood sugar levels to rise more quickly.

Examples of starchy vegetables to limit include:

- Potatoes
- Corn
- Peas
- Squash

Instead, choose non-starchy vegetables like leafy greens, broccoli, cauliflower, and green beans.

Processed Meats

Processed meats, such as bacon, sausage, and deli meats, are rich in salt and may have added sugars, making them unsuitable for a low-glycemic diet. These meats may also be linked to an increased risk of certain health problems such as heart disease and cancer.

Instead, choose lean protein sources like chicken, turkey, fish, tofu, and beans.

Bottom Line

A low-glycemic diet may provide several health advantages, such as better blood sugar management, enhanced heart health, and weight reduction. You can help to maintain stable blood sugar levels throughout the day and promote overall health and well-being by avoiding or limiting highly processed foods, sweetened beverages, high-sugar fruits, starchy vegetables, and processed meats. Concentrate on complete, minimally processed foods that are naturally low on the glycemic index, and supplement with lean protein and healthy fats.

CHAPTER 7:

FOODS TO EMPHASIZE ON A LOW-GLYCEMIC DIET

Concentrating on foods that are naturally low on the glycemic index and may assist in maintaining stable blood sugar levels throughout the day while following a low-glycemic diet is critical. These meals are often rich in fibre, protein, and healthy fats, which may aid in decreasing carbohydrate absorption and minimizing blood sugar rises. This book will examine some items that should be prioritized on a low-glycemic diet.

Non-Starchy Vegetables

Non-starchy veggies are strong in fibre and low in carbs, making them a good option for a low-glycemic diet. These veggies are also high in vitamins, minerals, and antioxidants, which may benefit general health and wellbeing.

Non-starchy vegetable examples to emphasize include:

Spinach, kale, and arugula are examples of leafy greens.

Broccoli, cauliflower, and Brussels sprouts are examples of cruciferous vegetables.

- Bell peppers
- Tomatoes
- Cucumbers
- Zucchini
- Asparagus
- Green beans

Including a variety of non-starchy veggies in your diet ensures that you obtain various nutrients and fibre.

Whole Grains

Whole grains are high in fibre and may aid in decreasing glucose absorption, making them a good option for a low-glycemic diet. Whole grains, as opposed to refined grains, which have been stripped of their fibre and nutrients, retain the bran, germ, and endosperm, making them a more nutritious option.

Examples of whole grains to emphasize include:

- Brown rice
- Quinoa
- Bulgur
- Barley

- Whole-wheat bread and pasta
- Oats

When selecting whole grains, check the label to ensure they are whole grains, not just "enriched" or "refined."

Lean Protein Sources

Lean protein foods such as chicken, fish, and tofu may aid in reducing carbohydrate absorption and minimize blood sugar rises. Protein is also necessary for muscle mass maintenance and growth, which may enhance metabolism and support weight reduction.

Examples of lean protein sources to emphasize include:

- Chicken breast

- Fish like salmon, tuna, and cod

- Turkey breast

- Tofu

- Beans

- Lentils

Regarding protein sources, consider lean cuts of meat and plant-based protein sources wherever feasible.

Healthy Fats

Good fats in nuts, seeds, and avocado may aid in decreasing carbohydrate absorption and improve satiety, making them an essential element of a low-glycemic diet. These fats may also aid in improving heart health and reducing inflammation in the body.

Examples of healthy fats to emphasize include:

- Nuts like almonds, walnuts, and pistachios

- Seeds like chia, flax, and pumpkin seeds

- Avocado

- Olive oil

- Fatty fish like salmon and sardines

When adding healthy fats to your diet, pick unsaturated fats such as those found in nuts, seeds, and fatty fish, and limit your consumption of saturated and trans fats.

Bottom Line

A low-glycemic diet may provide several health advantages, such as better blood sugar management, enhanced heart health, and weight reduction. You may assist in maintaining stable blood sugar levels throughout the day and enhance overall health and wellness by prioritizing non-starchy veggies, whole grains, lean protein sources, and healthy fats. Include various items in your diet to ensure that you receive various nutrients and fibre.

CHAPTER 8:

MEAL PLANNING AND RECIPES FOR A LOW-GLYCEMIC DIET

Following a low-glycemic diet requires careful meal planning. By planning and preparing meals, you can guarantee that you are consuming low-glycemic-index foods that will help you maintain stable blood sugar levels throughout the day. In this book, we'll look at some meal planning suggestions for a low-glycemic diet and some great meals to try.

Tips for Meal Planning on a Low-Glycemic Diet

Emphasize Non-Starchy Vegetables

In a low-glycemic diet, non-starchy veggies should form the basis of your meals. Strive to include a variety of veggies into your meals, and aim for at least two servings of vegetables at each meal. Leafy greens, broccoli, cauliflower, bell peppers, and zucchini are all excellent alternatives.

Choose Whole Grains

Choose whole grains that are high in fibre, such as quinoa, brown rice, whole-wheat bread and pasta. Avoid refined carbohydrates like white bread and white rice, which may promote blood sugar increases.

Include Lean Protein Sources

Lean protein foods such as chicken, fish, tofu, beans, and lentils may aid in reducing carbohydrate absorption and minimize blood sugar increases.

During each meal, aim to incorporate a dish of protein.

Add Healthy Fats

Healthy fats, such as those found in nuts, seeds, avocado, and olive oil, can help to slow carbohydrate absorption and promote satiety. During each meal, try to add a modest dose of healthy fats.

Make a Plan

Preparing ahead of time is essential for success on a low-glycemic diet. Spend some time each week planning your meals and prepping your supplies. This may help you save time over the week and avoid eating unhealthy, high-glycemic snacks.

Low-Glycemic Recipes to Try

Quinoa Salad with Roasted Vegetables and Feta Cheese

Ingredients:

- 1 cup quinoa, rinsed
- 2 cups water
- 2 cups chopped mixed vegetables (such as bell peppers, zucchini, and eggplant)
- 2 tablespoons olive oil
- 1/4 teaspoon salt
- 1/4 teaspoon black pepper
- 1/4 cup crumbled feta cheese

Instructions:

Preheat the oven to 400°F.

Bring the quinoa and water to a boil in a medium saucepan over high heat. Lower to low heat and cover for 15-20 minutes until the quinoa is soft and the water has been absorbed.

Meanwhile, stir the chopped veggies with olive oil, salt, and black pepper in a large mixing dish. Place the veggies on a baking sheet in a single layer and roast for 15-20 minutes or until soft and gently browned.

Combine the cooked quinoa and roasted veggies in a large mixing basin. Serve with crumbled feta cheese on top.

Baked Salmon with Asparagus and Brown Rice

Ingredients:

- 4 salmon fillets
- 1 pound asparagus, trimmed
- 2 cups cooked brown rice

- 2 tablespoons olive oil

- 1/4 teaspoon salt

- 1/4 teaspoon black pepper

Instructions:

Preheat the oven to 400°F.

Arrange the salmon fillets and asparagus in a single layer on a baking sheet. Add a drizzle of olive oil and some salt and black pepper, to taste.

Bake for 12-15 minutes, or until the salmon and asparagus are cooked through.

CHAPTER 9:

THE IMPACT OF HIGH BLOOD SUGAR ON HEALTH

Elevated blood sugar levels, commonly known as hyperglycemia, may have serious consequences for one's health. The human body requires glucose for energy, but consistently high blood sugar levels can lead to various health issues. This book will look at the effects of high blood sugar on health.

Type 2 Diabetes

Type 2 diabetes is among the most serious consequences of high blood sugar levels. Type 2 diabetes is a chronic illness that impairs the body's glucose metabolism. When blood sugar levels are continually high, the body may develop resistance to insulin, the hormone that aids in blood sugar regulation. This resistance may eventually contribute to the development of type 2 diabetes.

Cardiovascular Disease

Elevated blood sugar levels may also raise the likelihood of developing cardiovascular disease. When blood sugar levels are continually high, it may damage the blood vessels and arteries, accumulating plaque. This accumulation may cause artery narrowing, increasing the risk of a heart attack or stroke.

Kidney Disease

The kidneys remove waste from the body, but when blood sugar levels are continually high, the tiny blood capillaries in the kidneys may be damaged.

This damage may lead to renal disease or kidney failure in the long run.

Nerve Damage

High blood sugar levels may also result in nerve damage, known as neuropathy. Neuropathy is characterized by weakness and pain, as well as numbness or tingling in the hands and feet.

Eye Damage

High blood sugar levels may also damage the blood vessels in the eyes, resulting in various eye issues such as diabetic retinopathy, cataracts, and glaucoma.

Infections

High blood sugar levels may also damage the immune system, making the body's ability to fight infections more challenging. Diabetes makes people more vulnerable to infections such as urinary tract infections, skin infections, and gum disease.

Mental Health

High blood sugar levels may also influence mental health, according to research. According to research, high blood sugar levels have been linked to an increased risk of sadness, anxiety, and other mental health disorders.

How to Lower Blood Sugar Levels

Many lifestyle adjustments may assist in decreasing blood sugar levels and the risk of health issues.

Diet

A balanced diet is one of the most efficient strategies for controlling blood sugar levels. A low-glycemic diet, emphasizing foods low in sugar and carbs, may aid in blood sugar regulation and lower the risk of health issues. Non-starchy veggies, whole grains, lean protein, and healthy fats are good additions to a low-glycemic diet.

Exercise

Regular exercise may also aid with blood sugar regulation. Exercise improves insulin sensitivity, allowing the body to control blood sugar levels better. Aim for at least 30 minutes of moderate activity each day, such as brisk walking, cycling, or swimming.

Medication

Medication may be required in certain circumstances to assist in managing blood sugar levels. Type 2 diabetes may be treated with various drugs, including oral pills and insulin injections.

Stress Reduction

Since stress may affect blood sugar levels, it is important to handle stress efficiently. This might involve using relaxation methods like deep breathing or meditation, as well as receiving regular exercise.

In conclusion, excessive blood sugar levels may have a negative influence on general health, resulting in a variety of health issues. But, by implementing lifestyle changes, including eating a balanced diet, exercising regularly, and managing stress, blood sugar levels may be reduced and the risk of health issues reduced if you are worried about your blood pressure.

CHAPTER 10:

DIABETES: CAUSES, SYMPTOMS, AND MANAGEMENT

Chronic diabetes affects how the body utilizes glucose, the primary energy source for the body. Type 1 and type 2 diabetes are the two subtypes that are recognized.

This book will examine the causes, symptoms, and treatment of diabetes.

Causes of Diabetes

An autoimmune condition known as type 1 diabetes occurs when the immune system attacks and destroys pancreatic cells that produce the hormone insulin, which regulates blood sugar levels. While the precise origin of type 1 diabetes is unknown, it is thought to be a mix of hereditary and environmental factors.

Type 2 diabetes, on the other hand, is the result of a mix of hereditary and environmental variables. Overweight, sedentary people and those with a family history of diabetes are more prone to acquire type 2 diabetes. Type 2 diabetes develops when the body develops insulin resistance, increasing blood sugar levels.

Symptoms of Diabetes

Diabetes symptoms vary based on the kind of diabetes and the person.

Diabetes symptoms include the following:

- Increased thirst

- Frequent urination

- Fatigue

- Blurred vision

- Slow healing wounds

- Numbness or tingling in the hands or feet

- Unexplained weight loss (in type 1 diabetes)

- Management of Diabetes

Diabetes has no cure but can be properly controlled with the correct treatment strategy. Diabetes is normally managed with lifestyle modifications, medication, and frequent monitoring.

Changes in Lifestyle

Diabetes management may benefit greatly from lifestyle modifications. Among the lifestyle adjustments that may aid in diabetes management are:

Healthy Diet

A balanced diet is vital for diabetes management. A low-sugar, low-carbohydrate diet may assist in managing blood sugar levels and lower the risk of problems. A diet heavy in fibre, whole grains, and lean protein may also aid with diabetes management.

Regular Exercise

Frequent exercise may assist in enhancing insulin sensitivity, which can help the body control blood sugar levels more effectively. Aim for at least 30 minutes of moderate activity each day, such as brisk walking, cycling, or swimming.

Weight Control

Keeping a healthy weight is critical for diabetes management. Reducing weight may enhance insulin sensitivity and aid in blood sugar regulation.

Medication

Diabetes may be managed with a variety of drugs. These drugs affect blood sugar levels in various ways. Diabetes drugs that are often used include:

Insulin

Insulin is a hormone that controls blood glucose levels. People with type 1 diabetes typically need insulin shots to keep blood sugar levels under control. Some people with type 2 diabetes may need insulin injections if blood sugar levels cannot be adequately controlled by other medications.

Oral Medications

To assist in treating type 2 diabetes, a variety of oral medicines are available. These drugs affect blood sugar levels in various ways.

Monitoring

Diabetes management requires regular monitoring. Monitoring blood sugar levels may assist in spotting changes in blood sugar levels and allow for treatment plan modifications. Among the most prevalent monitoring approaches are:

Blood Sugar Screening

A glucose meter is used to assess blood sugar levels during blood sugar testing. Diabetes patients often test their blood sugar levels multiple times each day.

A1C Testing

The A1C test is a blood test that assesses three-month average blood sugar levels. This test is usually performed every three to six months to evaluate blood sugar levels.

Finally, diabetes is a chronic disease that alters how the body handles glucose. Type 1 diabetes is caused by an autoimmune reaction, while hereditary and environmental factors cause type 2 diabetes.

CHAPTER 11:

INSULIN RESISTANCE: CAUSES, SYMPTOMS, AND MANAGEMENT

Insulin resistance occurs when the cells of the body become resistant to the actions of insulin, resulting in high blood sugar levels. It is a leading cause of type 2 diabetes and other metabolic diseases. This book will examine the causes, symptoms, and treatment of insulin resistance.

Causes of Insulin Resistance

The precise aetiology of insulin resistance is unknown. However, it is considered a mix of hereditary and lifestyle factors. Some of the reasons that may lead to insulin resistance are as follows:

Obesity

One of the most important risk factors for insulin resistance is obesity. Excess body fat, especially abdominal fat, may contribute to insulin resistance.

Sedentary Way of Life

Sedentism may also lead to insulin resistance. Physical exercise regularly may assist in increasing insulin sensitivity.

Genetics

Some people may be predisposed to insulin resistance genetically.

Ageing

Insulin resistance may also worsen with age as the body's ability to use insulin declines.

Symptoms of Insulin Resistance

In the early phases of insulin resistance, there are often no symptoms. However, as insulin resistance worsens, it can cause a variety of symptoms, such as:

- Increased hunger
- Fatigue
- Difficulty losing weight
- High blood sugar levels
- High blood pressure
- High triglyceride levels
- Low HDL cholesterol levels
- Management of Insulin Resistance

Insulin resistance is normally managed with lifestyle modifications and, in some situations, medication.

Changes in Lifestyle

Lifestyle changes may help enhance insulin sensitivity and control insulin resistance. Among the lifestyle changes that can aid in the management of insulin resistance are:

Healthy Diet

A nutritious diet is critical for controlling insulin resistance. A low-sugar, low-carbohydrate diet may assist in managing blood sugar levels and prevent insulin resistance. A high-fibre, whole-grain, lean protein diet may also increase insulin sensitivity.

Regular Exercise

Frequent exercise may assist in enhancing insulin sensitivity, which can help the body control blood sugar levels more effectively. Aim for at least 30 minutes of moderate activity each day, such as brisk walking, cycling, or swimming.

Weight Control

Keeping a healthy weight is critical for insulin resistance management. Reducing weight may enhance insulin sensitivity and aid in blood sugar regulation.

Medication

Medication may be required in certain circumstances to address insulin resistance. Metformin is one medicine used to treat insulin resistance.

Metformin is a popular medicine used to treat insulin resistance. It works by lowering the quantity of glucose that the liver produces.

Insulin Sensitivities

Insulin sensitizers are drugs that aid in the improvement of insulin sensitivity. They function by assisting the body in making better utilization of insulin.

Other Medicines

To control insulin resistance problems, such as elevated cholesterol, other drugs, such as statins, may be recommended.

Finally, insulin resistance is a prevalent disease that may result in type 2 diabetes and other metabolic illnesses. It is caused by a combination of genetic and environmental factors and can result in various symptoms. Insulin resistance is normally managed with lifestyle modifications and, in some situations, medication. Improve insulin sensitivity and control insulin resistance through a nutritious diet, frequent exercise, and weight management.

CHAPTER 12:

HYPOGLYCEMIA: CAUSES, SYMPTOMS, AND MANAGEMENT

Hypoglycemia, commonly known as low blood sugar, occurs when the blood glucose level falls below normal. It is a prevalent disease caused by several variables, such as medicine, nutrition, and medical disorders. This book will examine the causes, symptoms, and treatment of hypoglycemia.

Causes of Hypoglycemia

Hypoglycemia may result from several circumstances, including:

Medication

Insulin and other diabetic drugs, as well as certain medications used to treat other medical disorders, such as beta-blockers, may produce hypoglycemia.

Diet

Hypoglycemia may be caused by eating too little or not eating enough carbs. Low blood sugar levels may be caused by skipping meals, fasting, or adopting a low-carbohydrate diet.

Medical Problems

Medical diseases, including liver disease, kidney illness, and insulin-producing tumours, may cause hypoglycemia.

Hypoglycemia Symptoms

Hypoglycemia symptoms vary from person to person, but frequent symptoms include:

- Shakiness
- Sweating
- Dizziness or lightheadedness
- Headache
- Fatigue
- Confusion or difficulty concentrating
- Irritability or mood changes
- Blurred vision
- Rapid heartbeat

Management of Hypoglycemia

Hypoglycemia is often treated by addressing the underlying cause of low blood sugar. Some hypoglycemic management techniques include:

Changing Medications

If hypoglycemia is caused by medicine, altering the amount or type of medication may assist with low blood sugar management.

Eating a Healthy Diet

Consuming a well-balanced meal with enough carbs may help avoid hypoglycemia. Having regular meals and snacks may also aid in blood sugar regulation.

Monitoring Blood Sugar Levels

Regular blood sugar monitoring may aid in the detection and management of hypoglycemia. Diabetes patients should constantly evaluate their blood sugar levels and alter their medicines and diet as appropriate.

Treating Hypoglycemia

If hypoglycemia develops, a fast-acting supply of glucose, such as juice or sweets, may be consumed to treat low blood sugar. Glucagon injections may be required in extreme situations.

Preventing Hypoglycemia

Avoiding hypoglycemia entails managing blood sugar levels and avoiding causes that might lead to low blood sugar. Some hypoglycemic prevention measures include:

Eating Regular Meals and Snacks

Eating regular meals and snacks may aid blood sugar regulation and prevent hypoglycemia.

Monitoring Blood Sugar Levels

Regular blood sugar monitoring may aid in detecting and managing hypoglycemia before it gets severe.

Changing Medications

If drugs are causing hypoglycemia, the amount or type of medication may need to be adjusted to avoid low blood sugar.

Staying Active

Frequent physical exercise may aid in the regulation of blood sugar levels and the prevention of hypoglycemia.

In conclusion, hypoglycemia is a frequent disorder caused by many variables such as medication, nutrition, and medical problems. Hypoglycemia symptoms might vary, but frequent ones include shakiness, perspiration, and dizziness. Hypoglycemia is often treated by addressing the underlying cause of low blood sugar, such as modifying medicines or eating a balanced diet. Taking precautions to maintain blood sugar levels is part of preventing hypoglycemia.

CHAPTER 13:

THE ROLE OF EXERCISE IN BLOOD SUGAR MANAGEMENT

Blood sugar control is an essential part of staying healthy. Too high or too low blood sugar levels may cause various health concerns, including diabetes, cardiovascular disease, and other chronic illnesses. Regular physical exercise is essential to any healthy lifestyle and has an important role in blood sugar regulation.

As you exercise, your body wants additional energy, which it gets by breaking down and utilizing glucose (sugar) in your blood. This procedure aids in the reduction of blood sugar levels, which is especially significant for those with diabetes or pre-diabetes. Regular exercise helps enhance insulin sensitivity, which means that your body is better able to utilize insulin to manage blood sugar levels and lower blood sugar levels.

Exercise can reduce fasting blood sugar levels, one of its most important advantages for control of blood sugar. After an overnight fast, fasting blood sugar readings give a snapshot of your body's blood sugar levels at rest. Elevated fasting blood sugar levels are a crucial symptom of insulin resistance, which, if addressed, may develop into diabetes. Even a single session of moderate-intensity exercise may considerably decrease fasting blood sugar levels in adults with or without diabetes, according to research.

Exercise can also enhance glucose tolerance, a significant advantage for blood sugar control. The capacity of your body to manage blood sugar levels in response to a meal is called glucose tolerance.

When you consume anything, your blood sugar levels increase as your body digests and absorbs the food. This mechanism, however, is interrupted in patients with diabetes or pre-diabetes, resulting in elevated blood sugar levels after meals. Frequent exercise may help your body balance blood sugar levels after meals by improving glucose tolerance.

Regular exercise may offer various health advantages and aid blood sugar control. It may assist in enhancing cardiovascular health, decrease inflammation, and promote mental health and wellness, for example. It may also aid in maintaining a healthy weight, which is essential for lowering the risk of diabetes and other chronic illnesses.

There are a few things to bear in mind when including exercise in your blood sugar control program. To begin, it is critical to choose activities that you love, and that are long-term sustainable. This might range from walking, cycling, swimming, or participating in a sport. Strive for 150 minutes of moderate-intensity weekly exercise spaced out across multiple days. Your regimen may also include strength training activities to enhance muscle mass and insulin sensitivity.

Before beginning a new fitness regimen, if you have diabetes or pre-diabetes, consult with your healthcare physician. They can assist you in developing a safe and successful workout plan tailored to your specific health requirements and objectives.

In conclusion, exercise is integral to any healthy lifestyle and important in blood sugar regulation. Physical exercise regularly may help reduce fasting blood sugar levels, enhance glucose tolerance, and improve insulin sensitivity. It may also improve cardiovascular health, reduce inflammation, and improve mental wellness, among other things. You may assist in maintaining healthy blood sugar levels and lower your risk of chronic illnesses by including regular exercise in your regimen.

CHAPTER 14:

THE ROLE OF SLEEP IN BLOOD SUGAR MANAGEMENT

Sleep is an important part of general health and wellbeing. Several physiological systems, including blood sugar management, rely on it. Poor sleep quality and quantity may interfere with the body's capacity to manage blood sugar levels, leading to various health issues such as diabetes, cardiovascular disease, and other chronic disorders. In this book, we will look at the significance of sleep in blood sugar regulation and the necessity of obtaining a good night's sleep.

The body goes through various physiological activities when sleeping, including managing blood sugar levels. Sleep deprivation may result in insulin resistance, a disease in which the body's ability to utilize insulin to control blood sugar levels is impaired. Insulin resistance may result in excessive blood sugar levels, which can contribute to type 2 diabetes development.

In addition to insulin resistance, insufficient sleep may cause alterations in appetite-regulating hormones such as ghrelin and leptin. Ghrelin is an appetite-stimulating hormone, while leptin is an appetite-suppressing hormone. When we don't get enough sleep, our ghrelin levels rise while our leptin levels fall, which may increase hunger and overeating. Overeating may lead to weight increase, a major risk factor for diabetes.

Sleep has also been proven to impact the body's capacity to react to stress. When stressed, our bodies produce stress chemicals like cortisol, which may raise blood sugar levels. A good night's sleep may help decrease stress, which can help control blood sugar levels.

So, how can you increase the quality and quantity of your sleep to help regulate your blood sugar?

Here are a few tips:

Keep A Regular Sleep Schedule: Try to go to bed and get up at the same times every day, including on the weekends. This may assist in regulating your body's normal sleep-wake cycle.

Make A Soothing Sleeping Environment: Ascertain that your bedroom is dark, quiet, and chilly. To block off light, consider employing blackout curtains or an eye mask. To shut out sounds, use earplugs or white noise.

Stimulants Should Be Avoided: Caffeine, nicotine, and alcohol should be avoided before bed since they may interfere with sleep quality.

Regular Exercise: Exercise regularly may assist in enhancing sleep quality and managing blood sugar levels. Nevertheless, avoid exercising too close to night since it might make falling asleep difficult.

Limit Screen Time Before Bed: The blue light generated by electronic gadgets might interfere with sleep. Avoid using electronic gadgets for at least an hour before going to bed.

Use Relaxing Techniques: Deep breathing, meditation, and yoga may all assist in decreasing stress and enhancing sleep quality.

In addition to these suggestions, it is important to consult with your healthcare professional if you are experiencing difficulty sleeping or regulating your blood sugar levels. They may assist you in developing a customized strategy that considers your specific health requirements and objectives.

Finally, sleep is important for blood sugar control, and poor sleep quality and quantity might impair the body's capacity to regulate blood sugar levels. You may help your body's capacity to manage blood sugar levels, lower your risk of diabetes and other chronic illnesses, and enhance your general health and wellbeing by boosting the quality and amount of your sleep.

CHAPTER 15:

SUPPLEMENTS AND HERBS FOR BLOOD SUGAR CONTROL

Keeping good blood sugar levels is essential for general health and happiness. Supplements, herbs, and a healthy diet and exercise may help with blood sugar management.

This book will look at various vitamins and herbs that aid blood sugar regulation.

Chromium: Chromium is a mineral that aids the body's utilization of insulin. Using chromium supplements has been found to enhance blood sugar management in persons with type 2 diabetes.

Alpha-lipoic acid: This antioxidant may help decrease inflammation and improve insulin sensitivity. Using alpha-lipoic acid supplements has been demonstrated in studies to aid in improving blood sugar management in persons with type 2 diabetes.

Cinnamon: Cinnamon has been demonstrated in studies to enhance insulin sensitivity and reduce blood sugar levels. Studies have demonstrated Cinnamon supplements aid in improving blood sugar management in persons with type 2 diabetes.

Gymnema Sylvestre is a plant used for ages in traditional Ayurveda medicine to help manage blood sugar levels. Gymnema sylvestre supplements have been found in studies to aid in improving blood sugar management in persons with type 2 diabetes.

Bitter melon is a vegetable often used in traditional Chinese medicine to help manage blood sugar levels. Using bitter melon supplements has improved blood sugar management in persons with type 2 diabetes.

Fenugreek is a herb traditionally used in Ayurveda medicine to help manage blood sugar levels. Studies have demonstrated Fenugreek pills aid in improving blood sugar management in persons with type 2 diabetes.

Berberine is a chemical found in various plants, including goldenseal and barberry. Studies have found Berberine supplements to aid in improving blood sugar management in persons with type 2 diabetes.

It should be noted that vitamins and herbs should not be taken instead of professional medical treatment or medicine recommended by a healthcare practitioner. Before beginning any new supplement or herb regimen, consult your healthcare professional, particularly if you use drugs or have any underlying health issues.

Apart from vitamins and herbs, you may do several additional lifestyle modifications to promote good blood sugar management. Here are some examples:

Eating A Nutritious Diet: A diet high in whole, unprocessed foods and low in added sugars and refined carbs may aid in blood sugar management. Regular exercise may help enhance insulin sensitivity and control blood sugar levels.

Stress Management: Prolonged stress might lead to elevated blood sugar levels. Relaxing methods such as deep breathing or meditation may reduce stress.

Obtaining Enough Sleep: Sleep is necessary for blood sugar management. Each night, aim for 7-8 hours of decent sleep.

Finally, vitamins and herbs may help to maintain appropriate blood sugar levels. But, before beginning any new supplement or herb regimen, consult with your healthcare physician, particularly if you are using drugs or have any underlying health issues. Making lifestyle adjustments such as eating a nutritious diet, exercising frequently, managing stress, and getting enough sleep, in addition to vitamins and herbs, may assist optimal blood sugar management.

CHAPTER 16:

ALTERNATIVE SWEETENERS AND THEIR IMPACT ON BLOOD SUGAR

Alternative sweeteners have become popular as people seek healthier alternatives to traditional sugar. These sweeteners are often touted as being lower in calories and less likely to cause blood sugar levels to rise than regular sugar. This book will look at some of the most popular alternative sweeteners and how they affect blood sugar levels.

Stevia: The leaves of the stevia plant are used to make stevia, a natural sweetener. It has grown in popularity recently due to its low-calorie content and little influence on blood sugar levels. Stevia has been demonstrated in studies to assist persons with type 2 diabetes in decreasing their blood sugar levels.

Erythritol is a sugar alcohol often used in low-calorie meals and drinks as a sugar alternative. It has a low glycemic index, which means that blood sugar levels are not greatly raised by it. It has also been shown that erythritol has little to no influence on insulin levels.

Xylitol: Another sugar alcohol that is commonly used as a sugar substitute in low-calorie foods and beverages is xylitol. It has a low glycemic index and does not raise blood sugar levels much. In addition, xylitol has been demonstrated to have little to no influence on insulin levels.

Monk Fruit: Monk fruit is a naturally occurring sweetener from the monk fruit plant. It has grown in popularity recently due to its low-calorie content and little influence on blood sugar levels. Monk fruit has been demonstrated in studies to assist persons with type 2 diabetes in decreasing their blood sugar levels.

Agave nectar is a natural sweetener made from the sap of the agave plant. It is often touted as a healthy alternative to sugar, yet it contains more fructose than ordinary sugar. This implies that excessive quantities might have a harmful influence on blood sugar levels.

Honey: Honey has been used for generations as a natural sweetener. Although it has certain health advantages, it is rich in calories and may influence blood sugar levels. According to research, honey may induce a greater spike in blood sugar levels than ordinary sugar.

Although alternative sweeteners may have less of an influence on blood sugar levels than normal sugar, they should still be used in moderation. Overusing any sweetener, including low-calorie or natural sweeteners, may result in weight gain and other health problems.

You may make various additional lifestyle adjustments in addition to utilizing alternative sweeteners to assist in good blood sugar management. Here are some examples:

Eating A Nutritious Diet: A diet high in whole, unprocessed foods and low in added sugars and refined carbs may aid in blood sugar management. Regular exercise may help enhance insulin sensitivity and control blood sugar levels.

Stress Control: High blood sugar levels may be exacerbated by chronic stress. Relaxing methods such as deep breathing or meditation may reduce stress.

Obtaining Enough Sleep: Sleep is necessary for blood sugar management. Each night, aim for 7-8 hours of decent sleep.

Finally, alternative sweeteners may be an effective strategy in promoting good blood sugar management. To enhance general health and wellness, it is vital to take them in moderation and adopt lifestyle adjustments like eating a good diet, exercising frequently, managing stress, and getting enough sleep.

CHAPTER 17:

THE FUTURE OF BLOOD SUGAR MANAGEMENT

Blood sugar control has advanced significantly in recent years, with new technologies, research, and therapies on the horizon that have the potential to alter the way we manage and prevent illnesses like diabetes. In this essay, we will look at some of the most recent improvements in blood sugar control and speculate on what the future may bring.

Continuous Glucose Monitoring (CGM): CGM is a device that enables people to monitor their blood sugar levels in real-time, 24 hours a day, seven days a week. A tiny sensor is implanted under the skin

112

and continually checks glucose levels, sending data to a receiver or smartphone app. CGM technology has already revolutionized diabetes treatment by enabling people to make more educated choices regarding diet, exercise, and medicine based on their current glucose levels. Smaller, more discrete sensors that may be worn for longer periods, as well as developments in data processing and interaction with other health technologies, are anticipated to characterize the future of CGM.

An artificial pancreas is a closed-loop device that combines a CGM sensor with an insulin pump to provide automated insulin administration in response to changing glucose levels. Clinical studies have shown encouraging results for this technology, with certain devices accessible in the United States and Europe. The artificial pancreas's future is anticipated to include more complex algorithms, interaction with other health technologies, and extension to incorporate additional hormones such as glucagon.

Smart Insulin is a novel form of insulin that responds to changing glucose levels, lowering the risk of hypoglycemia and improving glucose management. Researchers are actively investigating several ways to generate smart insulin, including nanotechnology and genetic engineering. Smart insulin, which is currently in its early phases of research, has the potential to improve diabetes treatment by offering more accurate and individualized insulin delivery.

Gene Therapy is the process of modifying the DNA of cells to cure or prevent illness. In blood sugar control, gene therapy might fix genetic flaws that cause illnesses like diabetes. Researchers are investigating several gene therapy options, including gene editing and substitution. Gene therapy, which is still in its early phases of research, has the potential to give long-term, curative therapies for diabetes and other illnesses.

Artificial Intelligence (AI): AI is a fast-evolving science with the potential to change healthcare in various ways, including blood sugar control. Artificial intelligence (AI) may be used to evaluate huge volumes of data from sources such as CGM sensors and electronic health records, offering insights and predictions regarding glucose management and the risk of complications. AI may also be used to create tailored treatment regimens and forecast the efficacy of various medications.

The future of artificial intelligence in blood sugar control is anticipated to include increasingly complex algorithms, interaction with other health technology, and extension to encompass additional health issues.

Nutrigenomics: The study of how diet influences gene expression and health consequences is known as nutrigenomics. Researchers are presently investigating how individualized dietary treatments based on genetic information might aid in preventing and managing illnesses such as diabetes. It may be able to build individualized nutrition regimens that help enhance blood sugar management and lower the risk of problems by examining an individual's genetic composition and eating habits.

The future of blood sugar control is bright, with several technological, scientific, and therapy breakthroughs on the horizon. Several promising breakthroughs have the potential to alter how we prevent and treat illnesses such as diabetes, ranging from CGM and artificial pancreas technology to gene therapy and AI. Although these developments are still in their early phases, they promise a future in which blood sugar control is more accurate, individualized, and successful. As research advances, many more fascinating innovations may probably emerge in the coming years.

CHAPTER 18:

MYTHS AND MISCONCEPTIONS ABOUT THE GLUCOSE REVOLUTION

Many myths and misconceptions about blood sugar management have arisen due to the glucose revolution, which describes the shift toward more glucose-friendly diets and lifestyles. This book will examine some of the most popular misunderstandings and falsehoods about the glucose revolution.

Myth: Carbohydrates, in general, are harmful to blood sugar regulation.

One of the most common misconceptions about blood sugar management is that all carbs are negative for blood sugar control. Although certain carbs, such as those in sugary beverages and highly processed meals, may produce fast blood sugar rises, not all carbohydrates are equal. Complex carbs, such as those found in whole grains, fruits, and vegetables, are broken down more slowly by the body, causing blood sugar levels to increase more slowly. Concentrating on selecting high-quality carbs rather than avoiding them entirely is vital.

Myth: If you have diabetes, you can't eat sweet things.

Another common misconception about blood sugar management is that people with diabetes cannot consume sweet foods. Although sugary meals may produce quick jumps in blood sugar levels, numerous other sweeteners can be used in moderation. Natural sweeteners like stevia and monk fruit have minimal to no influence on blood sugar levels, making them excellent substitutes for standard sweeteners like sugar.

Myth: To control blood sugar levels, you must avoid all fats.

The widespread belief is that all fats are detrimental to blood sugar regulation. Although certain fats, such as trans fats, may be hazardous to health, others, such as unsaturated fats in nuts, seeds, and avocados, can regulate blood sugar. Adding healthy fats to your diet may help slow down carbohydrate digestion and absorption, resulting in a more gradual increase in blood sugar levels.

Myth: Exercise has little effect on blood sugar regulation.

Many individuals feel that exercise is not necessary for blood sugar regulation. However, this is not the case. Physical exercise regularly may assist in improving blood sugar management by enhancing insulin sensitivity and stimulating glucose absorption into muscle cells. Exercise is widely regarded as one of the most effective strategies to improve blood sugar management and lower the risk of problems linked with diseases such as diabetes.

Myth: Blood sugar levels may be regulated only by food.

Although nutrition is crucial in controlling blood sugar levels, it is not the sole component. Additional lifestyle variables that influence blood sugar control include exercise and stress management. Those with diseases such as diabetes may also need drugs and insulin treatment. Working with a healthcare professional to develop a comprehensive treatment plan that addresses all aspects of blood sugar management is critical.

Myth: You don't need to test your blood sugar if you feel fine.

Another prevalent misconception is that blood sugar monitoring is unnecessary if you feel great. Many people with conditions such as diabetes, on the other hand, may not experience symptoms until their blood sugar levels have reached dangerously high levels. Frequent blood sugar monitoring is required to monitor glucose management and detect any problems before they become serious.

Finally, the glucose revolution has raised several myths and misunderstandings concerning blood sugar control. It is critical to distinguish between reality and fiction and to collaborate with a healthcare expert to create a complete treatment plan that includes all areas of blood sugar control. Individuals may improve their blood sugar control and lower the risk of problems associated with illnesses such as diabetes by concentrating on a balanced diet, regular exercise, stress management, and appropriate medication.

CHAPTER 19:

LIVING A LOW-GLYCEMIC LIFESTYLE: TIPS AND STRATEGIES.

A low-glycemic diet may improve blood sugar management and lower the risk of consequences from illnesses like diabetes. The glycemic index measures how rapidly a meal increases blood sugar levels, with high glycemic index foods generating swift spikes and low glycemic index foods causing delayed rises. This book will examine several tactics and recommendations for maintaining a low-glycemic lifestyle.

Focus On High-Quality Carbohydrates.

Selecting high-quality carbs is an essential part of maintaining a low-glycemic diet. Whole grains, fruits, vegetables, and legumes are high-quality carbs. The body breaks down these nutrients more slowly, resulting in a slower increase in blood sugar levels. It is critical to avoid highly processed meals and sugary beverages, which may induce blood sugar rises.

Incorporate Healthy Fats And Protein Into Meals.

Adding healthy fats and protein into meals may help reduce carbohydrate digestion and absorption, resulting in a slower increase in blood sugar levels. Nuts, seeds, avocados, and olive oil are healthy fats. Protein-rich foods include lean meats, fish, poultry, eggs, and lentils.

Be Mindful Of Portion Sizes.

Blood sugar levels may be significantly affected by portion size. It is important to keep portion sizes in mind and to strive for a balanced meal that contains a variety of carbs, protein, and healthy fats. Portion control may be improved by using smaller dishes, quantifying servings, and avoiding distractions when eating.

Choose Low-Glycemic Sweeteners.

Selecting low-glycemic sweeteners may help satisfy a sweet appetite while avoiding blood sugar increases. Sweeteners with a low glycemic index include stevia, monk fruit, and erythritol. It is important to use these sweeteners sparingly since they might still add to calorie consumption.

Incorporate Physical Activity Into A Daily Routine.

Physical exercise regularly may assist in improving blood sugar management by enhancing insulin sensitivity and stimulating glucose absorption into muscle cells. On most days of the week, aim for at least 30 minutes of moderate-intensity exercise. Brisk walking, cycling, and swimming are all excellent possibilities.

Manage Stress Levels.

Stress may impair blood sugar regulation by causing the production of hormones that elevate blood sugar levels. Finding healthy strategies to handle stress, such as practising relaxation techniques, getting adequate sleep, and participating in pleasant activities, is critical.

Plan Meals And Snacks.

Preparing ahead of time for meals and snacks may help guarantee that a low-glycemic diet is both maintainable and pleasurable. Experiment with new recipes, try new foods and combine different tastes and sensations. It's also good to have nutritious snacks such as nuts, seeds, and veggies to avoid overeating and blood sugar rising.

Monitor Blood Sugar Levels Regularly.

Those with diabetes should test their blood sugar levels regularly. Monitoring blood sugar levels may help uncover possible problems before they become a problem and help people change their treatment plans as needed.

Finally, adopting a low-glycemic diet may improve blood sugar management and lower the risk of problems linked with illnesses such as diabetes. Individuals can live a healthy and enjoyable low-glycemic lifestyle by focusing on high-quality carbohydrates, incorporating healthy fats and protein into meals, being mindful of portion sizes, choosing low-glycemic sweeteners, incorporating physical activity into daily routine, managing stress levels, planning meals and snacks, and regularly monitoring blood sugar levels. Collaborating with a healthcare practitioner to build an all-encompassing treatment strategy is critical.

CONCLUSION:

The Glucose Revolution has caused a substantial change in how we perceive and regulate blood sugar levels. The significance of maintaining good blood sugar levels in supporting general health and avoiding chronic illnesses such as diabetes has been underlined by this approach.

The Glucose Revolution has given people the skills and resources they need to take control of their blood sugar levels and adopt good lifestyle behaviours, thanks to science, technology, and education advances. The Glucose Revolution has prepared the way for a new era of blood sugar control, from discovering novel drugs and therapies to promoting a low-glycemic diet and frequent physical exercise.

There are still obstacles and misunderstandings about blood sugar control. Therefore, it is critical to continue teaching people about maintaining appropriate blood sugar levels and the tools for doing so. Sleep, vitamins, and alternative sweeteners are just a few examples of areas where more study is required to understand their influence on blood sugar levels properly.

The Glucose Revolution has made considerable progress in encouraging appropriate blood sugar management and providing people with the necessary skills and resources to take charge of their health. As we learn more about blood sugar regulation, we must be educated and make intentional choices about our lifestyle patterns too. We can continue to support the Glucose Revolution and live healthier, more meaningful lives by adopting a low-glycemic diet, including physical exercise into daily routines, and collaborating with healthcare specialists to establish a thorough treatment plan.

Printed in Great Britain
by Amazon

22672530R00075